HIDDEN HAND

A Cancer Book to End All Lies

By HENRY L. N. ANDERSON,
Ed.D., Ph.D., D.D., LL.D.

Henry L.N. Anderson

Enigami & Rednow Publishers, New York.
ISBN: 1-945674-10-5
ISBN-13: 978-1-945674-10-5

DEDICATION

To honor you, granddaughter Brianna K. Keaton, on your twenty-fourth birthday. May you share a creative, productive life.

AUTHOR'S PREFACE

This Small Book is sincerely dedicated to each individual who personally has been told; or who has been close to someone you know who has endured; and to everyone who is at risk of being devastated—one day, unexpectedly—by a medical practitioner who announces: 'You have terminal cancer, and there is nothing we can do.'

I also memorialize those who are no longer with us, some of whom who cradled their hysteria and their mental anguish—even their contempt and anger—because they painfully came to realize that 'they either could not afford what it was costing them, or they controlled too much wealth to remain alive....'

My deepest dedication prayer—in this Small Book—is that somehow, its essential message manages to survive distracters and finds its way into the hands, minds and lifestyles of those who are now 10, 20, 30, 40, 50 years removed from a potential 'day of personal terror!'

Finally, I dedicate this to Bernard Jensen, Ph.D., who declared miss-education and the deliberately orchestrated misguidance and misinformation of the people to be criminal behavior; and once again to Agnes Alberta Fox Anderson, my late wife of 36 years and 3 months whose 1975 breast cancer 'went away and returned' in 1993. My question, 'Where did it go?' should tell every woman—everyone, actually—there is a larger truth; and you, too, should strive to know it.

And, as Dr. Jensen stated it, 'to all others who have labored to awaken mankind to the knowledge that man's foods must be whole, natural and pure to sustain life at the wonderful level of health that Nature and Nature's Creator intended.'

Henry L. N. Anderson, B.S.Ed., M.A.R., Ed.D., D.D., Ph.D.,
Litt.D., LL.D., L.H.D., Th.D.

CONTENTS

ACKNOWLEDGMENTS

First of all I wish to pay humble respect to and show passionate gratitude for the willingness of friends and family who struggled with but, nonetheless shared their most terrifying and desperate 'disbeliefs.' Of course I am referring to their psychological trauma and their uncontrollable emotional breakdown that resulted, for each one of them, in its own unique fashion. The words I use to describe the contents herein belong to those to whom I make reference.

Historically, I am grateful to my three children who continue to support my speaking out about their mother's long and fatal connection to the 'cancer culture in American society.' It was her story that gave impetus to *The Nature and Purpose of Disease* (2001). I also thank my little brother, Clarence who has always been there for me, in so many different ways. And, this Small Book would not have been written but for the long-time friendship I have had with Tom Burke, who called me up one day and said, simply: 'Henry, are you at home? I need to talk to you!' This book is my answer to Tom.

In both instances my rhetoric was similar, pointed, and consistent with the science of healthful living, or Natural Hygiene, as best as I could articulate it. And for that limited capacity to express and share what I believe to be the fundamental truths associated with our God-given privilege to live a long, happy, and healthy life, I want to acknowledge several mentors and ideological 'ancestors' who made *the truth* knowable.

Dr. Herbert M. Shelton, Dr. Vivian Virginia Vetrano, Dr. T. C. Fry, Dr. John H. Tilden, 'Gypsy

Boots,' Marilyn and Harvey Diamond, Sarah Martel, Ken Desrosiers, Dr. Bernard Jensen, Dr. Alvenia Fulton, Dick Gregory, Dr. Aris La Tham, Dr. Nathan Rabb, Dr. Paul Goss, Dr. Joyce Willoughby, Dr. Bob Owens, Rudy Gerren, Dr. Eve Allen,

Dr. Tosca Haag, Victoria Bidwell, Dr. Margie N. Johnson, Dr. Thom L. Holmes, Stenson Tolan, Leonard Robinson, Gary Ricketts, Wintress and Don Barnes, and others like Mother Teresa in Calcutta, India and Rev. Dr. Martin Luther King, Jr. in New Haven, Connecticut, plus others, are acknowledged for their input, and guidance, and mentoring, and questioning, and even doubting my level of understanding. I acknowledge them, individually, and thank them collectively and immensely.

I am truly grateful to all the warriors who continued to challenge the establishment perspectives and push people toward knowing what is really true, however glossed up our common reality is made to appear. As I acknowledged Dr. Peter Duesberg and the many others who assert the 'HIV/AIDS' impossibility, I now lock hands with those who know that the path from the common cold to terminal cancer is the same path of our diets: what we eat, think, and drink, and how we manage our organic machines. We are resolute in our convictions. *We know prevention is the only 'cure.'*

EXCEPTIONAL AND RARE GREETING

From a Person who would have turned 103 on April 14, 2017.

Dr. Vivian Meador Johnson retired as a maternity ward LVN, beginning her studies at age 52 and retiring at age 83.

"Greetings! My name is Vivian Meador Johnson of Tyler, Texas. I was born on April 14, 1914 (will be 102 yrs old in 2016, God willing). Dr. Anderson is my son-in-law. He is 20 yrs my junior, but he thinks his book describes how I lived to be 101+ yrs old; with no pain; no problems; never been in a hospital; and am still grooving to Al Greene, especially on 'Love and Happiness!'

"I join Dr. Anderson in encouraging you to:
  1) be good to yourself,
  2) to respect everyone,
  3) eat right, two meals a day,
  4) to exercise daily; do some kind of movement.

Season's greetings,
Dr. Vivian Meador Johnson (Doctor of Humanities/Honorary Award).

Note* Dr. Vivian Meador Johnson expired on 12/30/2015 at the age of 101 years, 8 months, and 15 days). May she enjoy Eternity.

PREFACE

If you have been advised that your recent medical examination/analysis 'doesn't look too good,' or '…is not too encouraging,' or '…confirms your condition is terminal,' you don't have to tell me how that made you feel! I do understand. I understand a lot more than you might think. So, first off I want to share some of what I understand.

One, I understand—as do you—that no one lives forever; we all live for a limited time frame. We all know this, too. What we don't know, generally, is when we might die. Nor are we generally troubled by this lack of knowledge. But, we are all troubled by the issue of 'pain management,' at any time in our lives.

Two, I understand there is some kind of 'Natural Law' that holds humans responsible for their behaviors. Let me explain. If I drive my automobile in an irresponsible manner, I am more likely than not to cause serious injury—or even death—to myself and/or to others. So, I would have played a significant part in creating my own demise…or the demise of other, innocent persons. This relationship speaks to 'the law of cause and effect.' It would be just as true if the signal light (which someone invented to control traffic) malfunctioned and you and I lost our lives as a consequence of a head on collision.

Three, using the above examples, where injuries resulted, no one could predict the recovery index for each injured person. Individual differences and individual variability would come into play. In other words, the rate of healing or the level of healing—or the failure to heal—is unpredictable and uncertain, and will always be different from one person to another.

Four, whatever happens to us that is not yet fatal—will generate a variety of possibilities. While much might be dependent upon our physical conditioning, a significant importance must be given our mental state. Put differently, what we believe to be true...what we believe to be our 'situation' is 'critically linked' to what will truly become our situation.

Five, whatever (philosophy, belief, orientation, perception, pre-conditioning, 'mind control') sets the ticking of the mental clock...whoever wins the battle to control the mind...that slant will determine (more times than not) the perspective, the substance, the perception—the reality—that defines the individual condition or diagnosis. In other words, '...as a man thinketh, so is he....'

Six, given all of the predictors, medical science or science of healthful living notwithstanding, the diagnosis or the assessment could and can be in error. People given up on do live; people pronounced 'dead' have resumed life; and medical and scientific literature is replete with accounts of 'terminal' pronouncements being wrong. A UCLA study, for example, in 1985 reported that as many as 'nine out of ten diagnoses of cancer were in error.'

Seven, in the human timeline, there is a 'point of no return.' We all know that. What we don't know is when or where that point on the line is lodged. Given the best mental attitude and the worse physical conditions, persons have defied predictions and have continued to live productive lives. Also, given poor mental attitudes and what seemed quite 'treatable' conditions, people have just closed their eyes and died.'

Eight, once any human condition is declared to be 'critical'—whether the declaring voice is the 'terminal diagnosis' of the medical establishment or the 'crisis of toxemia' of the science of healthful living—only one of the two methodologies offers 'a true remedy.' I believe with all of my heart and mind that Natural Hygiene holds the real promise. That remedy—as I stated earlier—is prevention, about which I will say more later. Yet, some people survive medical treatments, and some do not 'come back' to good health pursuing Natural Hygiene.

Nine, I must state the exceptions. Where one follows the culture of establishment medicine, there are instances when outcomes defy projections. And, of course, this is true in instances where those involved adhered to and believed in the science of healthful living. Both disappointments and recoveries occur, and they cannot be reliably predicted. These 'unexpected' consequences are 'the exceptions.'

Ten, if you have not done so, use this occasion to: 1) Write out, record or otherwise dictate your 'Final Wishes;' 2) Clarify and make known 'the legacy' you wish to memorialize your love and life; and 3) Be comfortable that all your affairs are in order, and are properly spelled out. Your Will and/or Trust instrument should reflect your current and final wishes.

FOREWORD

What Are We Talking About? Before jumping on any given platform of critical conjecture or blissful platitudes, I wanted to review the boundaries of our co-existence. Being reminded of what we all must deal with can only help shape the substance and form of any campaign we might discuss to combat whatever it is we fear, fight, or favor. We are talking about facing your reality—and mine—head on, not overlooking any of what is real.

By now, perhaps, you are comfortably aware that I hold to a particular point of view relative to the issues and realities you and I will no doubt share. Whether I am right or wrong will not always be clearly discernable. Your views are important to me, but they are critical to your interests and concerns. My sharing with you what I would do, in your situation will be outlined, in detail. But, at the outset you are reminded that all that we say and do is co-dependent, coming from what we think we know and what exists beyond our knowledge. So, at a significant level of conscious awareness, you pray for God's mercy (always trying hard to think positive, remain faithful, believe strongly, hope fervently, and fight the battle to control what images your mind entertains!).

The expected response is to interface with your primary physician, then with 'specialists' to whom you are referred. And, you want to believe and to trust what you are advised; and you believe and cooperate in the decision making concerning what care you concur with.

Let me now speak with you in as gentle a fashion as is humanly possible. Let me say, first, that I love you—

not because we are friends, or because a friend sent you to me; not because we are relatives or members of the same social group, or because you have observed things about me over a period of time. I love you because you are a human being and as a child I was taught I should love my fellow human beings. So, I love you for no meritorious reasons of your own. My loving you is something that happened over a long period of time.

Consider at this moment what is most present in your mind, most urgent in your brain, most dear to your heart; consider your wildest wish, your strongest fear, your greatest prayer, and in so doing remember one thing: Whatever is your greatest concern is something that happened over a long period of time. Whether, as Natural Hygiene would describe it, you are now experiencing 'a crisis of toxemia,' or whether, as conventional medicine would describe it, you are now experiencing 'a terminal cancer,' it is something that took a long time to happen. The message here is very simple: your 'condition' did not just happen over the last few days or weeks or months or years; and, however it is described, this 'condition' will not disappear over the next few days or weeks or months or years....

What assurances can you glean from the above clarification? None, perhaps, except for the fact that whatever your mind perceives is the most likely actualization that will occur. Now, there is power in this juxtaposition. You are beginning to feel it. Continue feeling it, until you know it...deep down inside: in your stomach, in your guts, in your urine, in your thoughts, in your sleeping, in your breathing, in your laughing. Yes, in your laughing. Laughing.

Laugh; laugh a lot. Find more and more ways to laugh; find more and more situations that bring you laughter. Laugh like hell, like laughing suddenly became 'a religious exercise.' Do it as you remember your happiest times on earth.

In between laughing, try to forgive yourself for all your misdeeds throughout your early childhood, your teen years, your young adulthood, your adult life; work hard to convince yourself that you truly forgive yourself for past transgressions—against any and every 'feeling' person or creature on God's good earth. And, if there is someone or something you 'just cannot forgive,' pray to your God that He—or She—forgives you…and has mercy upon you, upon your soul…. You want your 'sin' (affliction, 'disease,' fear) to disappear (to be forgiven). That can happen, but you must first open the door through which 'forgiveness' (remission) must pass. If you cannot forgive yourself or another, you cannot 'receive forgiveness.' You are 'The Master' of your fate.

You can be helped to see from different angles, by hinting, by suggestion, and even by insinuation. You can practice 'looking into your mirror of life.' You can clean out your private 'closet,' where you have stored many valuable items; and no one else can open that door, or force you to open it. You hold the key, the key that is necessary to give you any real chance of upstaging that 'monster in your mind.' Misguided or false hope can be fully fueled with psychic poison, and no 'miracle' can be permitted to occur. This can happen despite 'the rule of exceptions.'

INTRODUCTION

Dearly Beloved, become kind to yourself. Embrace who you are now; and try very hard to at least 'like' the person that you are. Do not remain angry at yourself. Forgive yourself. You have been asked; so, do so. Do it now; do it soon; forgive yourself, as the premium you pay for the privilege of your healing prayer.

Declare your preference—that premeditated refusal or inability to forgive 'whomever' or whatever is so well stored in your mind and heart. You have the God-given right to think it might be okay, either way; but, as has been suggested before, you cannot be certain. Can you? Can you be certain…of anything? No doubt a "double blind study" would show that persons who refuse to forgive themselves, or others, also "refuse" to recover, even where recovery is not even close to the "point of no return." Free yourself of this possibility; forgive that part of your past. Embrace this prayer as a measure of hope and as a testimony to your acceptance of the Way of the Universe. Pray with me: *Great and Good Power of Your Creation, I close my eyes so that I might see eons more of your vast Universe, and so that I can feel a much better understanding of our dependence upon your Mercy, Protection, Patience, Blessings, and all your Goodness to us, without our deserving such consideration. Lord of the Universe, God of the mysterious One-Ness I thank you, for all of us, for your tolerance, for your BIGNESS (which we cannot comprehend); but we know because You allow us to exist. At the lowest place in our lives, at the loneliest moment of low self-esteem and rapidly declining belief or hope, we come, throwing ourselves before your feet, begging for Your Mercy. I have done wrong; we have done wrong. We have not been taught that which is right; and, where we might have been taught, we did not and have not learned; and we have lived wrongly. We have violated The Universal Rule, the Divine Law. We have not done the things required of us, which would have guaranteed us the Blessings we now seek. In this hour of affirmation, this time of facing up to What Is Real for Me—for us—please grant me—us—the vision that comforts and allows us to smile. Great "Unmoved Mover," as St. Thomas Aquinas dubbed Your Eminence, Thank you for allowing me/us to share in Your Creation. In appreciation of all that you have done for me, I now pray only that I be helped to rest my final concerns with Your Grace and Purpose…for me. Amen.*

Your mission is deeply personal; because you believe the 'stakes' are extremely high. But, in reality what you have is a distorted perception of your overall reality. There are critical connections—the 'juxtapositions' repeatedly referred to—which you have not fully understood; have not fully acknowledged; nor have you fully accepted. You are partially in denial. You also wish—if necessary—to "pull a rabbit out of the hat." You want to "escape the inevitable," if at all possible: to re-write the contract, or write an entirely new contract; to do whatever can be done to forestall this "critical status" which has become your mental burden. And, you have come seeking assistance, comfort, and understanding—even companionship—at "this eleventh hour." At this time, especially, you want, need, and expect to hear what is positive, what encourages hope. Yes, such assistance is awfully valuable to you at this emotional time. Based upon study and observation, coupled with replicated experience hope is embedded deep within the conviction that the Natural Hygiene amelioration strategies—if followed to the letter—will deliver the desired results. The odds favor the Natural Hygiene methodology. It becomes clearer that the creative genius of the human organism, *equipped as it is with the only healing power that exists*, will adapt to the corrective behaviors which Natural Hygiene teaches, demonstrates, illustrates, facilitates, articulates, and even orchestrates. There is one thing it cannot do; and that is all important. It cannot compel, force, or make you embrace and execute the requisite 'behavioral modifications.' You are the star player; you must do the dance to experience the romance. Are you ready? Are you truly ready to get started—or to continue in earnest? **Then, Let's Do It!**

What we can and will accomplish together should humble your spirits, inspire your neighbors, and confirm your faith in the principles and precepts of Natural Hygiene, the science of healthful living. And, in anticipation of the grace and goodness, we acknowledge the blessings we inherit from those crusaders ahead of us: Dr. Herbert M. Shelton, Dr. Vivian Virginia Vetrano, Dr. John H. Tilden, Dr. T. C. Fry, Dr. Alvenia Fulton, Dr. Nathan Rabb, Dr. Doug Graham, and many others such as Dr. Paul Goss, and even Dr. Sebi. We thank God for the simple truth, and for the wisdom to recognize and follow that truth.

What can be simpler? We must stop the poisoning. We must radically, as best we can, and as advisable, reduce the poison level. And, we must 'flood the organism with organic nutrients' and hygienic behaviors, beliefs, surroundings, activities, expectations, mental attitudes, exercises, relaxation, fun and enjoyment, peace and tranquility, excitement and laughter. Together, we must "do the right things." Separately, you must engage positive thinking and the recommended hygienic behaviors.

Now that I have taken you through a short overview of the philosophy and practice of the living science of Natural Hygiene, and while those impressions are continuing to form images in your mind—most of which will be constructive, and will contain 'healing properties'—I want to share a more global perspective concerning your personal matter which you have brought to my attention, seeking my input, counsel, assistance, and even my prayers—not to mention "any magic" I might bring to the table! And, we will come back to **specifically programming your life toward maximum and most urgent detoxification** (lowering the "level" of internal poisoning or toxemia), while radically ingesting organic nutrients, inculcating hygienic behaviors, and re-affirming our overall understanding of Natural Law and the 'mystery of life.'

1: IN THE BEGINNING

Most people would probably agree that everything that **is** had a beginning. But, it is hard to say how people would express what they envision about that beginning--the beginning of the universe. And, no matter how comfortable or how satisfied an individual might be with his or her view of that universal vastness, there most likely is a serene sense that all that vastness exists according to some fixed structure, law, rule, or order. Without some 'rule of law' that governs the whole of existence, 'destruction' would have long ago terminated existence, and we would not be here…most probably.

It is important to see and understand the 'absolute' premise that our lives are tied to a structured 'rule of law.' The clearer one's understanding of this connection between "life and the rule of life," the better grip one has on seeing the 'illusions and relativities' (misconceptions) about how the human organism navigates through 'the course of living.'

Suffice it to say that we are discussing a Rule of Law, and this law governs our lives to the fullest extent, and without exception; without partiality; without favoritism; without discrimination; without regard for personal idiosyncrasies. From the union of a 'small' sperm and a much larger 'egg,' a systemic 'law of living matter' embraces that union, never to let go again thereafter. The human cycle begins and ends consistent with universal law.

If our individual lives are controlled or governed by an absolute rule, doesn't it follow that we have no control over how our lives evolve? Isn't it equally true that we have no responsibility for how our lives evolve, or for what happens to us along the way? And, because this 'law of living things' as it applies to humans—to me, and to you—determines whether the egg is fertilized, in the first instance, and determines when we breathe our last breath, aren't humans victims of circumstances—no matter how you look at it?

The answers are Yes and No. Yes, we are victims, that is to say, we—each, individually—are unique. Of all the creatures that live, of all the humans alive—or that have ever lived, or will ever live, there never will be another you or another me. But, I would not classify that distinction as being a victim. I would call it a blessing: being created as a unique or very special individual!

To the question of whether we have control, responsibility, or say-so as to what happens with and to us as we evolve along the life line, I would say—absolutely—we do have all three! But, our control, responsibility, and say-so are not given to us alone, in isolation; it is given to us corporately, in concert with others in our environment. Some of what happens to us—consistent with the law of living—will happen because of the choices others make; and these outcomes affect us. We, ourselves, make the other set of choices which ensure—and prove—we are the 'other party' who determines our fate: the quality of our lives is determined by others, in concert with ourselves.

These are important lessons. The absolute characteristics of human existence are both our key to a quality existence and our guide for understanding the rules that lead to wellness or to illness, from little or none to a fatal amount. The control, responsibility, and say-so remain with us, whether we know it or not.

And, what we know—what we are encouraged to know—is controlled, largely by those who profit from our miss-education. There is a name for this; we call it *industrialization*.

I will give one example, not for argument sake but for illustration only. Why are humans the only living creatures who consume milk, after they are weaned? Could it be because humans are the only living creatures who manage a lucrative dairy industry? Do dairy products lead more toward human illness or toward human wellness? The answer you give reflects what you have been taught. Most of us were taught that milk makes a body strong, and is a great source of vitamin D and calcium. Real life evidence links milk to the build-up of mucous, the foundation of dis-ease. But what do you believe?

We live in a society which has taught us to depend upon the flesh of sea creatures, fowl, beef, pork, chicken, wild game, and even domesticated creatures as the best sources of protein for humans to consume. There is very little to remind us that The First Cause, the Unmoved Mover, God has put 'all the protein a human needs' in fruits, vegetables, nuts, and seeds (FVNS™). Nor are we told consumed flesh travels very slowly in the intestinal tract, taking three to five days to completely pass through, or longer depending upon conditions. This slow movement is costly because the flesh putrefies and produces poisonous gases and other chemical by-products. These gases pollute and compromise the body's operational systems (digestive, elimination, respiratory, circulatory, and lymphatic).

Industrialization requires a further look because it defines and describes the process we have referred to as "human evolution," the growth process that advances the human condition, leading mankind into higher levels of existence, i.e., electronic and mechanical structures, processes, systems, and overall internet co-existence.

We speak of our journey up from cave man to highly civilized and mechanized change agents; but we underplay our ancient superstitions and 'non-scientific' beliefs which define what we believe and how we rationalize the choices we make. And, this pattern of existence impacts every aspect of our lives.

Despite our level of sophistication as learned and evolving creatures, for reasons I cannot explain, we underplay our ancient superstitions, and how these impact current (and subconscious) impressions and basic or operational beliefs.

We prefer white people over people of color because in our fundamental makeup, we believe one person is better than the other, and that there is nothing wrong with preferring 'the better.' Is that what civilization and industrialization existence is all about? Many believe so. But why?

For example, why does 'society' hold onto its belief in the 'germ theory' of disease causation? Why does civilized humanity still believe one can 'catch a cold?' Or, why doesn't industrialized humanity not see the deadly correlation between meat eating (the consumption of all flesh) and the on-set of diabetes? And why do we ignore the clear connection between heart disease and the consumption of flesh foods? Heart disease is our number two killer, just behind cancer. Diabetes is third.

What is it that makes a society sane or wise? Would real-life correlations not be a major teaching tool?

Here is the point of this inquiry: as long as people can catch (somebody else's) cold they will not see the true dynamic unfolding before their eyes. All the true 'causes' (over indulgence, enervation, stress, excitement, depression, and fatigue), go unconnected.

In this state of what I will call 'ancient trans-phobia,' we allow ourselves to be victimized by bias and merchandizing, wherein we lose control of what we allow ourselves to believe and to act upon. In short, we are highly industrialized, and civilized victims of our own myopia. We succumb to the illogic, and are turned into victims controlled by pharmaceutical and medical merchandizers who generate 75% of all diseases.

2: THE LAW OF LIVING

Remember the 'law of living' that governs human existence, from beginning to end? What that law regulates might be referred to as 'equity.' If you do good, good will result; if you do bad, bad will result. If you consume an organic apple, for example, your body will receive the great benefits that come from eating the apple. By contrast, if you consume a hamburger, your body will receive the very 'stuff' that will add poison to your blood and 'liability' to the functioning of all your body's systems.

Let us pause a moment. Nothing said above is 'true' or 'false,' unless you believe it is either one or the other. You must take a position; and both statements cannot be true. Of course, you can say, 'But there is some truth, perhaps, in both statements.' Of course, you would be correct: what is true is relative to what one believes is true. Herein lies the 'rule of equity.' Garbage in equals garbage out.

If you consume good food and good beverages, your body will evolve in good ways; and if you feed your body foods that pollute, over the long term your body will show 'disease symptoms.' This is all consistent with 'the rule of equity' because we reap what we sow. We are not placing blame; we are recalling or reciting the 'Universal Law of Effects of Cause' (*Anderson, Nature and Purpose of Disease*, 2001).

By now it should be clear: certain behaviors beget wellness conditions, and certain other behaviors beget illness conditions. It is a hard and heavy dilemma, but you and I can win the battle of controlling what we consume, whether it is a plant-based diet or an animal-based diet, or even a modest mixture of the two. Your diet is everything you consume (food, drink, thoughts, beliefs, fears, hopes, and dreams) in the game of living your life. Nor should you ever forget: others are in businesses that profit from your negative behaviors, especially those behaviors that lead to critical illnesses and long-term dependencies upon drugs, chemicals, and procedures.

3: HOW MYSTERIOUS IS IT?

Are living and dying great mysteries to us? Do we linger in our thoughts about the source and possibility of life, of living? And, do we ponder the reality of death, or that everyone comes to that time when their lives end and they die? The phenomenon of life, or of death—how mysterious is either? No doubt you and I accept life and death; but, we have a question: What can I do if I am told, 'Your condition is terminal?' You can laugh like hell! Of course, your condition is terminal; it always was, remember? The Law of Living started out with us while we were a sperm seeking an egg; and it will remain with us through our last breaths. So, regarding the 'devastating pronouncement,' what can or what should you do in response to this diagnosis?

You can pray, and perhaps you should. You can seek second and third opinions, and perhaps you should. You can laugh, as we suggested earlier, at the 'surprise' character of the announcement, when you might have reminded the announcer that 'the rule' has not changed. 'Terminal' does not mean 'here today and gone tomorrow.' 'Terminal' means 'will end.' So, what is there that exists that is not terminal? I think you are getting the picture. Now you see why I am writing this all down. Too many have come, asking the same question, sharing the same pronouncement of doom!

Of course, my responses are different, but only because the individuals who come are different. What makes this 'little book' viable is that it contains my fundamental reply, my essential response. The 'Gestalt,' if you will, of my wholistic message is the same (thank God for the late, Wholistic Saint, Dr. Alvenia Fulton of Chicago, Illinois, the vegetarian who taught both Dick Gregory and me the fine art of therapeutic fasting). There is but one Truth; and that truth begs to be told, to be shared, to be ingested; to be known…and to be believed. Here's my test question: Do you want to live…?

4: RIGHT TO LIFE

Remember, through all of your life no one has ever questioned your right to life, liberty, and the pursuit of happiness. First it was your right to life; next it was your right to liberty; and finally came your right to pursue happiness. Pause here for a few moments. Now, consider this: someone, for whom you represent an unspecified sum of money, is expecting you to pay her or him, and for what? She or he expects to be paid for being the first person in your life to tell you to begin thinking about death and dying! Remember, 'Your condition is terminal?'

Let us not begin a quarrel. Let us not take this matter lightly. Let us remain calm, inquisitive, and unconvinced. And you should be all of these, and more. You should listen keenly and keep eye contact with the professional. You should reflect upon your diet over the most recent months and years. You should wait for her or him to tell you—from what she or he 'knows' about your organism—what might have brought her or him to the conclusion: 'Your condition is terminal.'

What you want to hear next is lay language, which non-medics can understand. You want to hear and/or see correlations. For example, if you have over the past several years eaten multiple meals in a week from any fast food chain, that should tell you something you heard earlier and already know, something about 'equity,' about 'what goes in must come out.' You understand, immediately, that if you have been long exposed to radiation in the workplace, or to environmental toxins in your residential community, or if you had military exposure to bio-chemicals, these are correlations that lead to maximum internal pollution. You need to hear such juxtapositions from the 'professional team' that has elected to turn your thinking toward death. Your ears want to hear connections between 'behaviors and conditions,' between 'input and output,' between 'causes and effects,' to the best of the professionals' ability to share their analyses with you. Short of these happenings, laugh—again—and pronounce: 'I will seek a second opinion and get back to you.'

Say you went through all of that already. Now, you are in the aftermath of up and down feelings, anxieties and confusion, tears and consternations, doubts and fears, some outrage and some anger—mixed feelings. You come to me, nervously, look me in the eye and ask: 'Can we talk? I need to talk to you....'

5: WHAT YOU TELL ME

Female, Age 61: My doctor told me the breast cancer I had 19 years ago has returned, and it has metastasized. He said it has spread throughout my system and I should put my affairs in order; I have maybe ninety days, he said.

Working together, and based upon my fundamental beliefs and total support of persons who confide in me, there was a period during which, her doctor told her: 'Your cancer is in remission; our treatment is working.'

The 'treatment' referred to by the doctor was the small pills (Tamoxifen) the size and shape of vitamin B-12 tablets, but slightly pink in color. The client declined to take the pills; so she was not 'under treatment,' as the doctor thought.

Nearly four years from the '90-day window' announced by her doctor, the client passed away, in the quiet of the early morning hours; and, she died of respiratory failure. For the last 15 months of her life, she was unable to breathe on her own. She was convinced she had made the right choice in following natural hygiene and she only wished she had made it much sooner in her life. When asked what she valued most in all of life, she responded: 'My husband....' She was my first wife.

6: WHAT I TELL YOU

Dearest Paula:

I am responding to your having received depressing, if not devastating input, presumably from medical personnel. These are my personal views, beliefs, and notions about the subject matter which tends to fill the psyche of both the person receiving the input/information and the person giving that same 'verbal gemstone.'

Because of you and others, what I am saying in this Small Book is 'absolute.' That is to say, I give my most personal response to the concerns inherent in the shocking news or devastating pronouncement. How any reader responds is up to that reader. But, here is what I believe—and given the same experience I would stake my life on—repeating what is revealed, immediately doing what is described; embracing the Natural Hygiene philosophy and lifestyle as the next best path...since "prevention" was obviously missed. Now, the task is to undo, turn back, reverse, or enforce 'remission.' First, the 'damning' behaviors must be stopped; and, next, the level of toxemia (systemic pollution) must be methodically reduced as quickly and as thoroughly as possible; and a number of support and complimentary behaviors must run concurrent to our first and second actions. These three...are the redeeming strategy, if any at all exists. Not only is living regenerative, but the body is already imbued with the only 'healing powers' available. This does not, however, make it possible for you to grow a new finger or toe!

What I am saying here—above—and throughout these presentments is, perhaps, too simple to be so profound: Disease by whatever name arises out of the vortex of internalized pollution, and is principally the by-product of industrialization. This means a great amount of "dis-ease" is inevitably generic to the evolving social order in which you live. Massive food production; gas-electric-petroleum energy supplies; transportation of people, marketing products by land, sea, and air; human and animal shelter and fresh water; waste management; and non-edible production of goods—all of these produce pollutants which humans ingest throughout their daily lives. This 'ingestion' cannot be prevented or eliminated; however, it can be mitigate when you understand this reality and implement the 'Rules of Wellness.'

7: MEASURES OF CONTROL

Furthermore, it is possible to regain the larger measure of control over your well-being. Your awareness of the 'internal pollution' theory empowers you; you can discover and embellish your behaviors which improve the human condition. You learn important—and now obvious—relationships between an act that you do and the consequence that action has on your state of being. And, even if you cannot see the immediate effect, you know that having just eaten a mango will produce more positive results than if you had just eaten a six-once fish steak.

More importantly, so long as you 'accept' the notion that when your body is out of sync and malfunctions, it is because you have 'caught a virus,' you are tied to 'ancient superstitions' and you give control over your life to a huge system, an industrialized sub-component known as 'the medical establishment.' Let us be clear; what we are talking about here is 'dis-ease' or mal-function of the human organism—what is commonly called illness, sickness, acute and chronic disease. We are not talking about accidents: broken bones, severed and bleeding flesh, child birth, systemic mal-function, and various emergencies. When you see this distinction, you also can see and respect the legitimate role of medical science within an industrialized, civilized, and socialized society. We do need medical doctors and associated professional staff.

This 'knowledge' we are sharing here is the only 'protection' you can have against that same medical establishment, that industrialized complex of people and processes whose companion objective is to produce capital, cash—profits! It is what Harvard

Researcher and highly respected scientific scholar, Dr. Charles Thomas, referred to as 'the *hidden hand*' that drives the increasing volume of money-making or cash-intensive 'diseases,' the largest of which—by far—is the so-called 'HIV-AIDS' paradigm (see T.C. Fry, *The Great AIDS Hoax,* 1987).

Don't get me wrong; I am not against medical science. However, I do reject three (3) of its fundamental precepts: 1) the viral cause of 'dis-ease,' 2) the theory of 'contagion,' and 3) that 'disease' is an entity or is various and sundry 'entities.' Natural Hygiene is so clear and logical when it shows the relationship between 'internal toxicity/toxemia' and 'symptoms of distress' within the body. This comparison or juxtaposition is easily tested and verified. For example, consume spoiled food and the body immediately reacts by vomiting, with diarrhea, by gagging, or even coughing, running nose or even skin irritations or discolorations. The different reactions are consistent with the individuality of the impacted bodies. My point, though, is clear: if you control the cause (ingesting spoiled foodstuff), you also control the 'effects' (symptoms), food poisoning. The major point is that the vomiting was not caused by your being exposed to a virus.

The rule also applies to what is known as 'the common cold.' You did not 'catch a virus,' or your neighbor's kid's cough; however, you did go without sufficient sleep; you ate something the body had not eliminated; you over indulged drugs or chemicals; you failed to get sufficient rest; you over-consumed simple sugar, caffeine, or other compounds; or you engaged a number of other 'high-risk' behaviors, including inhaling gaseous or polluted air (such as air exhaled by a person who smokes).

I could go on and on; but, remember this: Groups of people don't come down with similar symptoms except when they consume similar poisons, whether via air, water, food, beverage, or substances taken by mouth, including drugs, chemicals, herbs, medications or any combinations of these, and not to the exclusion of so-called 'athletic' or 'power' drinks. If you watch sports, no doubt you have seen, at the end of the game, the coach is doused with the left-over "Gator Ade." What you don't see is that the drink could be spiked, so coaching staff can add either 'stimulant' or 'depressant,' depending upon which behavior the staff wants. And, at the end of the game, the 'evidence' is 'destroyed' when it is poured over the coach's head! You saw but you did not see.

The process of living is filled with many 'illusions.' The literature is filled with reports of "outbreaks" which finally point to specific 'poison pockets,' not to 'caught viruses.' My late and beloved hygienic mentor, T. C. Fry, D.Sc. would have agreed that 'Persons exposed to similar 'causes' will show similar 'effects'.'

Male, Age 69: I wish I had changed my diet 20 years ago, as you advised me. I will never forget that you sponsored and invited some 200 people to a vegetarian dinner at that downtown hotel. Even though I know there was no meat served, in my mind that spinach pasta had chunks of 'meat' in it. And, I know it was not meat, but diced eggplant in the vegetable sauce. I know but my mind still sees meat.

If I had followed your advice, I probably would not have had my first stroke, then the next one; and my 'borderline diabetes' would not have escalated to the medicated condition I suffered over the years. I ate a lot of the wrong stuff—from old habits; but, I knew better. You and Dr. Fry explained the connection between how and what I ate and what might happen later in terms of health complaints. I did not see it, or did not believe it, or was just too into my lifestyle to see any reason to change it. I regret that now....

Is it too late...? I know I probably shouldn't even ask that, so I won't; let's talk about your disease book. There is something I've wanted to ask. How can disease have a purpose? You know, in your book title, *The Nature and Purpose of Disease*?

My Friend:

First, it is never too late to do the right thing. If an improvement in consumption is done, an improvement in consequences will result. This is consistent with what natural hygiene teaches. A better seed produces a better plant; a better plant renders a healthier food; and a healthier food contributes to a healthier organism, and this holds true weather it is animal or human who consumes the better food. Here's another example: if a pail is catching water from a leak in the ceiling and the pail fills up, there is spillage, right? But, if some of the content of the pail is removed, the drips from the ceiling fall into the pail without spilling. Two principles are illustrated here. One, it was clear that sooner or later the pail would fill; and to prevent spillage, an action to remove some of the content had to occur. Two, if the removal activity continued, conceivably that same pail could continue to catch drips far into the future. So it is with the human organism. It can collect and store pollution, in varying amounts and for various periods of time…before any 'spillage' occurs. So, I ask you: Is it ever too late to remove some of the content from the pail…allowing it to continue to catch drips?

Natural Hygiene postulates that 'disease' is not an entity or commodity, but a quantitative description. In other words, this thing we name for location and intensity is really a measurement, an indication of the level of storage, pollution, toxicity, poisoning, disruption, interference, rotting, cancer or decay within a living organism (animal or plant). What is seen is the 'evidence,' the symptom of this accumulated, now toxic preoccupation—the dis-ease, wherever it occurs.

The purpose served by the symptom, or by the particular 'crisis of toxemia' site is extremely important; it signals a problem, a threat to the survival of the organism. Humans respond to accumulating crises based on their location and level of intensity. If too much activity brings on a heart attack, the symptoms will be recognized by a knowledgeable observer. Furthermore, this heart disease is, itself, the consequence of accumulated toxic storage within the organism; and, over time the presence of all that poisonous stuff has compromised normal body function, and the 'victim' is one who did not alter her or his lifestyle soon enough to prevent the 'heart attack.'

The purpose of disease, then, is to communicate the relative status of wellness of this or of that organism. The reference, fundamentally, is to the level of body pollution, and where in the body the built-up is most probable. By sending this message, your body is telling you something needs to be done. That if left unattended to, the continued storage would cause more and more interference and disruption in how your body normally functions; and over a long period, these invasive levels will curtail normal life expectancy by causing the organism to malfunction or even to die prematurely.

What I am saying is Biology 101 or Life Science 100; it repeats what this book started out with, pointing out the absolute correlations between 'cause and effect,' between healthy intake and healthy output; between actions that are consistent with the rules and principles of healthful living and actions that result in the myriad names of unhealthy conditions that we call by all sorts of disease names. This Universal Law is so simple, yet so absolute; it does not matter whether you agree with it or not; whether 'scientific prognostications' confuse people into believing what is not true; or whether the evidence is not absolutely clear. But, here are simpler truths: 1) You will never die in a plane crash if you are never in touch with a plane. 2) You will not have watermelon seeds in your feces if you never consume watermelon. 3) You will not satisfy your craving for caffeine by eating fresh mangos. The point I am pushing here should be obvious; and, when it comes to the life-long and life-enriching benefits gained from consuming organic and raw FVNS™ (fruits, vegetables, nuts, and seeds), along with the wellness behaviors recommended by natural hygiene, you can expect healthful living and abundant wellness.

You have been told, also, what you need to do toward reversing any negative or non-productive pattern of living, or status of physical existence. To be sure, I am not referring to imperfections of nature, where a body does not function 'normally' because it was afflicted at birth or later. Nor am I forgetting injuries and maladies which might have occurred after birth, from whatever causes. Given all of the conditions and probabilities of 'normal living,' pursuing a healthful living lifestyle is protective and reassuring. Much of the decision process is subject to the temptations, early teachings and learning, and cultural influences that pervade the larger community, and the targeted and directed 'consumer messages' beamed at your mental receptacles by Wall Street (The Industrial Complex). Remember, internal pollution begins—in the present era—with the reality of and need for the industrialized character of contemporary, global co-existence. In short, the stuff of dis-ease is automatic; your goal is to control how much becomes a part of your act of living. And, when—and if—you learn your body is experiencing a 'crisis of toxemia,' this book is, hopefully, a guide to your best counter fight! *Use it to live.*

And while doing so, realize that 'famines in Africa' must be given to 'organized genocide' which result from starvation, unclean water, and hostile environments—all of which are preventable....

8: DO YOU WANT TO LIVE?

I must ask that question, first, because it is true that sometimes persons will not readily admit that they really 'don't want to be here anymore.' Whatever might be your political point of view is irrelevant. If a person wants to use her or his God-given 'choice' to conclude she or he no longer finds this life satisfying and wishes, as soon as possible, to 'not be here,' that is her or his right (but would be 'wrong' under the law, to terminate existence). But, you can assume any person who has come or will come to me for consultation, comes because she or he wants to live.

So, then, how do you live in the face of a devastating diagnosis? Very simply: you live as you always have, committed to what you believe in; and, if your belief structure needs tweaking, you tweak it. What do I mean by that? Obviously, if you had done everything 'right' during the course of your life, you would not now be seeking solace regarding this fearful and terrifying 'terminal' pronouncement. So, you face the fact that your 'diet' led you to your various stages of wellness, or lack thereof. Now, let me tell you what I recommend, and why.

9: THE SCIENCE OF HEALTHFUL LIVING

I am a follower of Dr. Herbert M. Shelton, Dr. Vivian Virginia Vetrano, Dr. T. C. Fry, pretty much in that order, all of whom deemed themselves 'Natural Hygienists.' Dr. Shelton was, perhaps, the principal researcher, writer, lecturer, and challenger of the conventional medical establishment. Dr. Shelton 'proved,' for example, that 'all disease was the same disease;' that disease was not an entity, but a quantitative symptom of a body giving notice that its normal functioning is being disrupted by 'foreign elements' within the system. Simply put, when collected poisoning disrupts body function, some physical sign or evidence is produced. Dr. John Tilden referred to this condition as 'a crisis of toxemia.' We can also call it internal pollution. That is why we encourage detoxification actions.

What if the medical professional's 'devastating pronouncement' were identical to the 'crisis of toxemia' described by Tilden, Shelton, Fry and others? One thing for sure: it would mean that both professionals saw similar evidence that an organism was in crisis, that a human entity was dealing with and adjusting to internal content that had compromised the integrity of the would-be healthier body. And both perspectives would be correct. Now something deliberate or 'radical' begs to be done. Only what they would recommend is as different as night is from day. The tools of the medical establishment are surgery, radiation, and treatments (using drugs, chemicals, and machines). The tools of natural hygiene are fasting, detoxification, wellness activities, and a raw diet (fruits, vegetables, nuts, and seeds...organically grown, and the juices of these), plus pure water (alkaline, preferably, because 'cancer' requires an acidic environment as research has indicated).

Subjectively considering the tools and philosophies of the medical establishment and those of the international natural hygiene movement, (www.OrganicWellnessCrusade.com © by HLNA, 1990), each person has to decide which 'Master' will be followed. The decision here is crucial; it is 'a life and death' decision. Remember, the medical professional first made the announcement: 'Your condition is terminal.' You 'laughed' at the pronouncement then; and you should 'laugh' at it now. You must make your decision; will your prescription be toward conventional medicine or toward traditional natural hygiene? I claim some qualification only on the natural hygiene side. Unless there is similar commitment to a 'science of healthful living' response, I can offer no advice and little assistance. I have little to do with medicines and drugs.

Here is what my friend, Dr. Bernard Jensen, of Escondido, California wrote several years ago: "We are committing a crime when we do not let people know that they are doing a serious wrong to themselves if they do not live a clean, healthful life insofar as it is possible in our civilized world of today. Failure to teach the public that they are producing bad tissue because of bad living habits, and keeping them from knowing that they are producing the soil for a possible cancerous growth as the result—should be considered a crime. Public education on the correct way to live has been neglected far beyond what it should be, and one of these days we will recognize this as our greatest need."

In 1931, Dr. Otto Heinrich Warburg won the Nobel Prize for discovering 'the real cause of cancer in 1923.' Why it took eight years for him to receive the formal recognition is not clear. Dr. Warburg was Director of the Kaiser Wilhelm Institute (later renamed the Max Planck Institute) for cell physiology at Berlin. He investigated the metabolism of tumors and the respiration of cells, particularly cancer cells.

What Dr. Warburg observed was that all 'cancerous tissues are acidic, whereas healthy tissues are alkaline!' He explained the finding by pointing out that water ($H2O$) splits into $H=$ and $OH-$ ions; and 'if there is an excess of $H=$, it is acidic; if there is an excess of $OH-$, then it is alkaline.'

Dr. Warburg established that 'all normal cells have an absolute requirement for oxygen; but cancer cells can live without oxygen—a rule without exception.' He further concluded that if cells are deprived of oxygen for 48 hours, they 'may become cancerous.'

His over-riding conclusion, which puts the spotlight on exactly what cancerous cellular status truly is, he states as 'oxygen deficiency (brought about by toxemia).' And, in later years, John H. Tilden, MD took up the mantle stating, with Dr. Herbert Shelton, that 'disease' (specifically and generally) represents 'a crisis of toxemia.' And, therefore, echoes Dr. Shelton, 'All disease is the same disease!'

Dr. Warburg further supported his conclusions by his discovery that 'cancer cells are anaerobic (do not breathe oxygen) and cannot survive in the presence of high levels of oxygen.' This should be enough—it should have been enough, even in 1923, for the medical establishment to structure a clearly articulated 'prevention program' for the protection of the general public. Instead, we have the massive 'cancer industry' which thrives at the expense of the general public, and is growing every year! *This, despite the New England Journal of Medicine declaring, in 1985, that after 30 years of 'cancer research,' the incidents of cancer continue to rise, leading to the conclusion that, 'The only reliable cure for cancer is prevention.' Prevention is also the key to removing cancer's 'cash value' underpinning, as Harvard researcher, Dr. Charles Thompson postulates.*

It is this 'hidden hand,' this hugely monetary aspect which 'feeds' the cancer industry. Not until the cash cow is put down will any noticeable decline become apparent. **Cancer is an industry, a complete, structured cash-generating economic system. It is highly sophisticated, jealously protected, and convincingly marketed. It manipulates its own best interests.**

What should a person do who has been diagnosed with cancer? This is an important question; and the answer is perhaps more critical than is the question. For the answer is dependent upon a good many variables: who you are, where you live, what you believe, what is your story, what has been your lifestyle, what is your belief structure, what is your financial position, what is your health (wellness) profile, what does your doctor say, what is your relationship with your doctor, how you feel and what you believe about your circumstances (including your physical condition), and other questions including to what are you committed, and what your views are concerning a raw, organic FVNS™ diet.

The consensus in this presentment is that acidosis is at the root cause of any bio-chemical cancer diagnosis: that any reversal of 'the effect' must implement an amelioration strategy that mitigates 'the cause.' The practical aspects of this construct are real; in fact, they are so valid and measurable that any success at lessening the concern will come only in direct proportion to the status of the condition in the organism. In other words, since the absolutely fool-proof 'cure'—prevention—was not employed, we are now at the mercy of all the specific variables that are present in the particular situation or diagnosis. That, notwithstanding, UCLA cancer researchers declared, also in 1985, that 'nine out of every ten diagnoses of 'cancer' are incorrect.' The numbers for petrol-chemical cancers will be different; and psycho-chemical cancers are virtually unacknowledged in medical literature. I would argue that more people die annually from 'cancers they believe they have' than from real 'cancerous conditions.'

Even so, when the pollution level within the organism reaches 'the crisis stage' it is a matter of extreme urgency, a time for 'radical action.' Whether one is responding to a diagnosis of cancer or an assessment of a crisis of toxemia, it is most likely an indication that much internal damage has already been done.

There is a message in this rendering; there are messages in this presentment. 'Hope' is hidden in here somewhere. My prayer is that you will find it....

10: ESTABLISHING CREDIBILITY

Persons who do not know me will want to examine my background, experience, published books, speeches, articles, lectures, public statements, formal education, and tutelage by my hygienic mentors, Dr. T. C. Fry and Dr. V. V. Vetrano, Sarah Martel, M.S., Dr. Richard Rosenbloom, and even Kenneth Desrosiers, Ph.D. and various members in the raw foods movement, especially Dr. Aris La Tham (guru creator of Sun Fired Foods™), Gary Ricketts (Los Angeles herbalist), Dr. Doug Graham, Dr. Nathan Rabb, Dr. Joyce Willoughby, Dr. Paul Goss, Dr. Cherilyn Lee, Dr. Eve Allen and numerous others.

In the final analysis, one who comes with a 'message of doom' must be self-motivated enough to examine the diabolical options, and make the choice that Natural Hygienists believe is the only credible choice. It is, as has been suggested, a life and death decision; it is ultimate; it is absolute; it is self-actualizing; Natural Hygienists believe it is the only path back from any abyss. Clearly, Natural Hygienists do not believe the 'prophets of doom.' Research has shown over and over that up to 9 diagnoses out of 10 have been wrong by the medical profession, especially regarding terminal conditions. And, believe it or not, there is 'a God Presence' active in the affairs of mankind.

Scientific progress has been dismal. The New England Journal of Medicine, May 8, 1986, summed up the dilemma, thusly: For more than thirty years, the medical profession has been 'losing the war against cancer.' Given all the research and treatment modalities available, 'the most promising areas are in cancer prevention rather than treatment.' We are, now, twenty four years from that announcement! So, over the last fifty-plus years, only Natural Hygiene has provided a winning option for those with concerns about ultimate predictions, announcements, or 'diagnoses.' Raw, organic food consumers seldom—if ever—face any cancer issues whatsoever. Vegetables are alkaline; animal products are acidic. Cancer strives in an acidic environment; but, cancer perishes in an alkaline environment. Petrol-chemical and psycho-chemical cancers manifest differently.

So, take a short break; make a bathroom call; breathe deeply and relax; and come back. Let's talk, specifically, to your concern. Let me tell you exactly WHAT TO DO.

11: RECOMMENDED BEHAVIORS
[Rules of Wellness]

Here is a list of good behaviors; do as many of them as you can, as often as you can:

- Eat only when hungry; but never over eat. Over-eating is dangerous and deadly.
- Eat enough to feel satisfied, not until you feel full.
- Drink no liquids immediately before, during, or after eating; liquids slow digestion and cause other concerns.
- Eat foods in proper combinations: fruits first, vegetables with proteins, starches with veggies. Do not eat protein foods (nuts, seeds, green vegetables) with carbohydrates.
- Seek out organically grown foods, fresh and raw; packaged in glass, not medal or plastic.
- Basically consume FVNS™ (fruits, vegetables, nuts, and seeds…raw and organic) and their juices (fresh squeezed, and consumed within ten minutes of juicing).
- Breathe fresh air, filtered air, purified air, unscented air, wholesome air.
- Eat "mono meals" (a meal of only grapes; apples; mangos; avocados; nectarines, etc.).
- Avoid processed foods, noted for salt, sugar, MSG and other chemical contents.
- Do not become "addicted to the good taste of bad foods" (as in sodas, candies, etc.).
- Chew one mouth full of food at a time, until it disappears, chewing 40-100 times. Do not

shovel food into your mouth, roll it and swallow. Un-chewed and unprocessed food generates fat & pollution.

- Do not use eating time for talking; digestive enzymes are in the mouth, where they need to mix thoroughly with the food in order to break it down for processing and distribution throughout the body.

- Eat organic, raw FVNS—the best foods on earth for humans; everything else is down hill.

- Enjoy ethnic and cultural foods (dishes) sparingly; you decide the frequency and the amount. Do not eat to satisfy another. Generally, "The cook outlives the person served."

- Drink alkaline water if available; next distilled, or spring; back off plastic bottled water.

- Consume mostly "frugetables"© (FVNS™, their fresh-squeezed juices and combinations).

- Exercise vigorously at least every other day; but do some 'workout' daily (in sunshine, fresh air, pleasant surroundings, and under peaceful and safe conditions—alone or with others).

- Treat your body like your "best friend," caringly and lovingly, always with respect.

- Pass the 'mirror test' regularly (look in the mirror and confirm aloud: 'I love you!').

- Rotate your choice of fresh, raw foods for the widest variety, consumed within 3 days of purchase.

- Forgive yourself; go all the way back, from childhood to the most recent time in your life.

And forgive others. You must give forgiveness to receive it.

- Live in a tranquil environment and attain peace of mind. Avoid stress levels by de-valuating (whatever it is).

- Do not consume food in a rush; it will not digest and will add to internal pollution/toxicity.

- Chew your smoothies--even your water; remember digestive enzymes are mostly in your mouth.

- Lose weight by "eating yourself thinner" (4-6 'small meals' of FVNS™ per day; only fruits after 8PM or within 2 hours of your bedtime. Eat fruits 24/7, melons first, bananas last.

- Eat dried fruit (non-sulfured) first, on an empty stomach; but never as a dessert.

- "Foods" that are not listed are not recommended (dairy, all flesh, caffeine, sodas, alcohol, drugs, herbs, cooked, pickled, canned, boiled, shelled, exotic, unknown, ancient), with exceptions based upon routine human intercourse and controlled consumption.

- Let your money buy the best food available on earth and your food will make your days long, upon this land which 'the Lord giveth thee.' And your food will be your 'medicine.'

- Increase laughter in your life; relax and always enjoy living.

- Learn how to do 'therapeutic fasting' (*The Nature and Purpose of Disease*, Ch. 17, p. 250) and do one fast every six months. Initially, just 3 days or so; later, with experience, as many as 21

days or more, depending upon your personal and/or wellness objective/s. Until you are very experienced and proficient, you should fast in consultation with a professional. Regarding all the information contained herein, which is offered for educational purposes, use it at your own discretion. Send questions or comments to dr.anderson@cula.edu, or visit the website:
www.OrganicWellnessCrusade.com.

- Pray, meditate or otherwise express your spiritual dimension, however you perceive that aspect of your life.

One who does not see a wellness path might want to become fat; fatty tissues are said to capture and isolate some quantity of pollution from the vital organs of the body.

12: FACING YOUR ULTIMATE PERIL

First off, if you believe you have lived a relatively clean, good, and healthy life, and you question strongly 'this panic announcement' you have been sent home with, there is but one thing to do: immediately reject the notion! Put it in the spam folder. You have to believe in yourself, in your own assessment of your physical condition. Because, at this moment, there is a battle being waged and that battle is about mind control. The person who gave you that 'devastating pronouncement' presumed to be in control of your mind. You were not asked for permission to be given that kind of fatalistic information. You were not warned that—given so many odds, etc.—there is some, slight possibility that 'our test results will show, will suggest...' No, the 'establishment person' just created an opening and laid it on you: 'Your condition could be terminal.'

However it was said, it had to be known that it would cause at least 'quiet panic' in your brain. The announcing physician found it necessary to first establish, going forward, who is in control of the scenario. You were put on the defensive; you were stripped of your option to object or to disagree—even to disbelieve. You were treated as a child who is handed a piece of candy. 'Oh, what a nice person!' Not, why would you hand a child a 'cancer stick?' What looked like a kind gesture was, in fact, one strike toward the final out. You must first come to this conclusion yourself; if in fact that is how you believe it to be.

Do you agree with the pronouncement, or not? If you do not agree, have you convinced your mind that you do not agree? Remember, your mind has been 'attacked…ambushed.' A different and deadly 'reality' has been 'created' in your brain. 'Your condition is terminal' rings like a loud church bell: ding dong, Ding Dong, DING DONG! And, you hear it, whether you want to or not. And you don't want to; that's why we are talking. That is why you wanted to talk to me. You know enough about me to believe I WOULD NOT HEAR THE DING DONG! Sure, you were correct. Now, we are together….

What I will say to you from this point on is going to be dubious. It will be dubious because my words—or the words of Natural Hygiene—are just words. They have little or no meaning until they are actualized by your behaviors; and your behaviors need their orders and instructions from your brain. And, remember, you are dealing with a 'damaged brain.' I am here to help you; but, you must be here to help me, too. I cannot tell you to believe, or to not believe. You must tell me…that you believe. And when you do, my heaven, we can 'turn water into wine!'

My first born child, Brenda, once asked me: 'Daddy, what is your purpose for living?' I thought about it and said: 'You know, Brenda, I believe my purpose for being here—for living—is to be at the right place, at the right time, to say the right thing, to the right person, in the right way, at the right moment….' She looked at me with a slightly brighter continence and replied calmly and with a bit of serenity: 'Dad, you do that all the time.' I said, 'Yes, I guess I do; so, I guess each time I do it, it means my purpose in life is to do it again!' We chuckled softly, and both felt a sense of profound enlightenment. We never had that issue come up again between us. No matter where in the world I go; no matter who from the far corners of the world I bring and invite to our home, it is expected, because that is who I am; that is my mission; that is why I am here...on this good earth. I am okay with that.

13: NOW, LET'S GET RIGHT DOWN TO IT

Considering what you have shared, I am okay with what you were told—even with your stampede, your 'devastation.' I know what is true. So, let me ask again: What do you want from me?

'I want you to know what I am feeling. I want to tell you my situation; and I want to know that I can confide in you; that I can share my concerns. And, I want you to tell me what you think I should do now. I know you; I trust you; I have observed you over the years and I have seen how you remain healthy and vibrant. I know I have not followed your lead; I have not pursued a disciplined lifestyle. There are many things I might have done, which I have not done. Now, despite that, I would like your support as I attempt to chart my course, from this moment on. If you will assist me in this, I will be grateful.

WHAT YOU SHOULD DO

Okay, I will tell you what you should do. 1. You should stop and give thanks, because your situation could've been worse. 2. Take a careful look at the word, disease. Does it tell you anything about itself? For example, do you see—in it—a 'statement of condition?' Do you see the DIS-EASE in the word? 3. What can you articulate about your 'critical' dis-ease? In other words, when you analyze your condition, your major complaint, your assessment of what went wrong, can you visualize what went wrong, and when it began to happen, and whether you ignored earlier 'warnings' or any tell-tale messages 'symptom message' your body (and mind) sent you from time to time? Can you admit—even if only to yourself—to the 'extreme behaviors' you indulged at earlier stages in your life? For example, 'binge drinking' (you know, those great youth parties, with all the alcohol, drugs, sweet-acidic-fast-foods, sexual activity, exposure to heat-cold-radiation-salt intake-oily snacks, ice-cream, candy, energy drinks, inadequate drinking water consumption?

4. Correlations emerge; and they are specific, real, and 'costly.' We know these 'effects of cause' as autism, dyslexia, 'crack baby,' bi-polar, retarded, hyper-active, deformed, mentally retarded, handicapped, 'special needs,' and other 'deformities' are correlated to 'binge behaviors' 10-25 years ago.

Some 'relationships' can never be seen with the naked eye. For example, you can watch a relative go in and out of hospitals for amputations of toes, feet, leg parts, sometimes fingers, and some even endure amputation of both legs. What is the central correlation, you ask? It is called 'flesh eating'. Human beings were to find their food in 'the garden of Eden,' not in the 'Cattle Ranchers Spread.'

Correlations guide our vision, that we might see the truth; illusions entertain us while we are 'blinded.' While we ponder family history, we credit daddy's brother, Frank, for my weak heart valve. My aunt Martha on my Mom's side was diabetic—and so was her younger sister. But, this cancer…I don't know where it comes from. Test yourself—and prove me wrong: find a diabetic who is not a meat eater. Or, a bad heart victim who is not carnivorous. Now, that brings us back to cancer (and cancer diagnoses). I will end this discussion with one admonition: take care what you believe because: In the history of the human race, no one has ever 'caught a common cold.' Cancer is preventable. Some 'cancers' are reversible; and some cancers are manageable…while there are 'cancers' that 'exist' only in the human mind.

So, let's take charge of this situation; let's show 'um!

14: GREAT! LET'S DO IT!

- Stop, or radically curtail polluting your body and mind.
- Reduce the level of retained toxicity.
- Consume a massive amount of organic, raw nutrients.
- Radically change behaviors to those recommended by natural hygiene.
- Engage exercise and physical fitness routines
- Learn therapeutic fasting; do one every six months
- Experience abundant laughter
- Maintain a positive mental attitude (mind-control)
- Do specified and monitored organs and system "cleansing"
- Self-forgiveness, forgive others, forgive your situation
- Embrace peace, quiet, warmth, acceptance, safety, sharing
- Read, study, question, require, demand, compromise, agree
- Keep to your own dream/s; but come to accept your 'reality'
- Give thanks…engage prayer /meditation; worship/contemplate
- Keep a note book, journal, tally, daily on-going record
- Weight and even height, skin coloration or texture
  - Special occurrences, notable events, mental or physical changes
  - Notable input from others

- Observations [in nature, people, sound, media, animals]
- Your thoughts and feelings, urges, cravings, wishes, dreams
- Count your blessings, over and over and over again and again
- Give thanks where thanks is due, and forgive yourself for sure
- Confess your love…for whomever, for whatever, for real
- Fret not, do not worry, be positive, be philosophical
- Fear not, marry your understanding with your reality
- Believe…believe…believe and trust what and who you believe
- Be prepared…for whatever evolves…until it comes
- Continue to share your joys…and even your fears [if any]
- Practice saying "thank you" to whomever, about whatever
- Make promises only to yourself … and keep them real
- You decide what you want going forward

Now, let's make it all happen! Let's just do it!

15: REDEMPTIVE ACTIONS

In the science of healthful living, redemptive action begins with the first taste of plant-based mother's milk. Exercise and recommended hygienic behaviors protect and nourish the evolving body-mind-spirit to maturity and beyond. In instances where habits and behaviors strayed off course, there were likely times when the organism experienced distresses, from what at the beginning point is called 'the common cold' and at the extreme other end, Herbert M. Shelton, ND and John H. Tilden, MD concurred was 'a crisis of toxemia.'

T. C. Fry, D.Sc. was my mentor and I believed what I learned through him, because it was so simple yet made so much sense—and answered so many of my tough questions. Dr. Fry admonished that 'sickness' or 'illness' was not 'natural,' in that it would not occur if the 'causal behaviors' were not engaged. And, later I learned that those causal behaviors came either from our own actions and/or from the actions of others.

Now, here you are; full of 'crisis, disease, and terminal illness.' What do you do? You pray; you hope that you have not 'come to your senses' too late to self-correct. You pray; you deeply wish you can reverse, or at least noticeably slow the motion toward premature death. After all, you still want to live, because you 'are not ready to die.' I understand; I do. Because I understand—and want to understand even more—I am writing this 'small book,' sort of as 'a guide of hope at any desperate time.'

First, I must confess: I believe your energy to reach out for another perspective is the evidence that feeds my belief that, as my mother used to say, 'As long as there is life, there is hope!' I believe that the combination of your will to live and my wish to confirm life, offers a clear path of Natural Hygiene as the 'corrective behaviors' of choice. Personally, I believe that if there is a path back from any abyss, it is the path of Natural Hygiene.

Second, I am absolutely convinced that the hygienic behaviors that follow are those that were recommended from the time of your birth. Doing them now cannot erase past experiences but surely can, and will retard further progression toward future crisis-disease-terminal illness. What is offered following is a win-win life option. Do it to live; do it to live longer. Do it because you want to win. Do it because you are smart. So, let's do it....

16: THE NATURAL HYGIENE, HEALTHFUL LIVING LIFESTYLE

- Stop the poisoning; do not poison yourself
- Reduce the level of retained poisons
- Consume abundant nourishment & exercise, body & mind
- Passionately engage hygienic behaviors 24 hours, seven days
- Study the science of healthful living; share learnings
- Live life at the edge, with much laughter & forgiveness
- Be thankful, be a wellness crusader, and be a missionary

17: STOP THE POISONING

The human organism takes in pollutants from the air, water, food, and thoughts that are encountered. Food is perhaps the most dominant source of internal poisoning. So, Natural Hygiene's principal 'treatment modality' is therapeutic fasting, that is abstaining from all food and beverage (except pure water) for a minimum of three (3) days. The art of fasting is a common experience; we do it over night and in the morning we 'break-the-fast' (breakfast) to start our day.

Abstaining from food, for therapeutic purposes, requires knowledge and skill; and fasting longer than three days should be conducted under the guidance of a trained and knowledgeable wellness professional. One to three-day fasting takes place in our lives frequently: when not feeling well; when too rushed to eat; when traveling; when dissatisfied with the menu options; when the atmosphere is not conducive to consuming food, and any number of other scenarios.

Fasting immediately stops adding pollutants from food as a source. Fasting also conserves vital energy resources by not having to expend for the processing of nutrients and the elimination of exposable and non-exposable stuff. This conserved energy is then re-directed by the organism and is used to clean out and neutralize retained toxins.

Taking in foods that require minimum processing—such as fresh-squeezed juices and smoothies—is the next closest act to fasting. Not everyone is able to engage therapeutic fasting, even a limited-day fast; but, juicing is second best and will not significantly alter the desired outcome.

As a part of any 'critical treatment modality,' there are some important guidelines for juicing and blending. For example,

Fresh squeezed juice (of one or more compatible fruits/vegetables) should be consumed within fifteen minutes of its extraction. A fruit juice should have 'a green' component, using kale, collard, cabbage, or other green and leafy plants.

Eating 'mono-meals' (consisting of one food, i.e., grapes or apples or mangos or avocadoes, or melons) might better serve those who must chew their meals. Natural Hygiene strongly encourages substantial chewing of all food, and even 'chewing' drinking water. The reason is simple: digestive enzymes are in the mouth; the act of chewing mixes these vital enzymes with the food, pairing them up—in a sense—for transporting this 'nutrient' content to all parts of the body. Why 'chew' water? It puts 'extra' enzymes in the stomach to better facilitate the processing of anything in the stomach that needs to be moved out. Interferon (the healing substance in the organism) is said to be produced only in an empty stomach. You are looking for healing.

18: REDUCE THE LEVEL OF RETAINED POISONS

You have strayed from your pre-ordained 'path to good health, long and happy life.' You have done so in too many ways to articulate. No matter; now, you must earnestly strive to reduce the level of toxic waste your body and mind have collected and stored over the years. Fasting, juicing, smoothies, mono-meals, and even alternate-day eating can help reduce retained toxicity levels.

More deliberate actions, generally referred to as detoxifying procedures, should be administered by trained professionals, whether it involves herbs, by capsule or tea or other forms; or colonics; or enemas; or purges; or sweats; or manipulations; or other internal cleansing strategies. You must remember—at all times—your condition today took a very long time to develop; it will take some time, also, to regress.

Every act of more positive thinking; of more invigorating laughter; of more relaxed and unstressed living; or more loving and nurturing environment; or more helpful and forgiving feelings and thoughts will increase positive karma and reduce the level of toxemia your organism carries daily.

I must admonish you—now:
DO NOT BLAME YOURSELF…for anything.
FORGIVE YOURSELF for everything.
And, YOU MUST FORGIVE EVERYONE ELSE (You know who they are!). This single act of forgiveness is critical to the success of your effort to make amends for your own past transgressions. Your body/mind would not be at risk had you not violated

many cardinal rules of 'the science of healthful living,' Natural Hygiene. Forgive, so that you can be forgiven.

19: CONSUME ABUNDANT NOURISHMENT & EXERCISE FOR BODY AND MIND

There is nothing on earth more valuable to you at this time—and at any time, really—than the acquisition and consumption of fresh, organically grown fruits, vegetables, nuts, and seeds (FVNS™). To acquire certified (and actual) organic foodstuff defies almost any pricing or distance limitations. In other words, there is nothing on God's Good Earth that is more valuable than the food you eat! 'Let your food be your medicine.'

The vegetarian lifestyle is embraced by Natural Hygiene because research of every kind and description, and researchers from every philosophical persuasion agree on one construct: the longer food remains within the digestive system, the more gases and chemicals are created and these extol a price, and that 'price' is increasingly high and extremely negative.

Flesh consumed by humans may not partially exit the organism for five to nine days, depending upon the particular organism; while plants could pass through that same organism in from minutes to hours, rarely taking more than one day.

There is no 'wellness' difference among fish, pork, beef, chicken (shell fish, other fowl or wild game, etc.) and other than fruits, vegetables, nuts and seeds, raw and organically produced and delivered to your table, everything else is downhill in the food chain. One of the worse 'other consumables' is, perhaps, the 'soft drink.' Its sugar, caffeine, and chemical contents cripple children and deprive adults of useful kidneys and other organs in their latter years. Soft drinks add poison content and also kill.

Exercise, yes exercise! Do some activities every day, in the name of exercise, recreation, and fitness—call it what you like; but, do it! Your body is a 'machine' with many moving parts; it has systems and sub-systems and all benefit from motion, resistance, cleansing activities and gauged tasking. Your body needs sunshine, fresh air, clean water, gentle touching, and times for rest and rejuvenation.

Your mind needs the same kind of special attention. In fact, it is more important to caress your mind, to cleanse it of 'stale stuff' than it is to reduce the level of toxins in the body. Toxins in the mind are more dangerous if they get out of control. 'As a man thinketh, so is he.' Remember, I said that earlier on. Now, hear this: As your mind believes, so your body achieves. You want to move back from 'crisis?' You want to see signs your body 'is fighting back?' You want to win the challenge your body is putting forth? Control your mind; let your mind tell you all will be well, following wellness principles.

20: PASSIONATELY ENGAGE HYGIENIC BEHAVIORS EVERY DAY OF YOUR LIFE

Let me ask you, how hard is it to eat fresh fruits and vegetables, not having to cook them? How difficult is it to munch on raw nuts and seeds, one handful at a time? Even if you soak them first, or blend them, or consume all of these in combinations that work, how cool is that? How convenient is it to reach into a handbag, briefcase, tote bag, or back seat and pull out a healthy snack—one or two pieces of fruits--even an entire meal?

If you can fill your life with live foods, alkaline water, and a lifestyle of 'fun and games' that are shared and cared for by an appreciating circle of mutually loving individuals, you would be as near to a 'heavenly' environment as is possible...on earth! If you can laugh—and cry; if you can laugh even more and cry even less; if you can either laugh or cry, you can live a quality life. Life is not measured by how long you live, but by how well you live. You know that so well. Can you really imagine what it is like feeling 'just great' every single day?

21: STUDY THE SCIENCE OF HEALTHFUL LIVING

Share What You Learn. If you learn the fundamentals of Natural Hygiene, you can 'fire your doctor.' Once you embrace the principles and precepts of 'the science of healthful living,' you will have guaranteed to yourself that you will be healthy and well, and can pursue happiness as a vocational choice, helping other people, making the world a better place, showing appreciation for and to those who blazed the trails that led to the simple truths that control our lives—those you are aware of, and those that stare at you and you do not see them. Once you know that no one ever 'catches a cold', you have been liberated, set free; and, you can now begin to live free—truly free (from the enslaving illusions of modern medicine, that system which 'encourages' a debilitating lifestyle). You would have re-captured control of your mind.

For starters, Google Herbert M. Shelton, John H. Tilden, Vivian Virginia Vetrano, T. C. Fry, Alvenia Fulton, Paul Goss, Bernard Jensen, Tosca Haag, Douglas Graham, Nathan Rabb and read some of the early history of The American Natural Hygiene Society. Do this; and take a break from your concerns about yourself. Trust Natural Hygiene as much as it trusts you. Make short visits to www.organicwellnesscrusade.com and smile.

22: BE THANKFUL, BECOME A WELLNESS CRUSADER, BE A MISSIONARY

Right now I feel like being prayerful: Almighty God I have come so far following the light which you shone. I pray I have not lost my way; I pray that I have followed as you directed. I pray that I have said what you told me to say, that I have learned what you wanted me to learn, and that I have been obedient and worthy of the task you put before me. Now, Father, with tears in my own heart I bow down before You and ask that You forgive my sins of humanity, that You excuse and forgive my errors and omissions, that You have mercy upon Your sons and Your daughters who are dealing with pain, both physical and mental, spiritual and historical, and to the memory of my dearly beloved mother, Dr. Louise Burns Lonon Anderson (1912-1992), I pray for your blessings...Amen.

Dearly Beloved, whoever you are who reads this, I love you as an Agent of the God of my beliefs. It is not important that I know your name, or your face, or your circumstances, or that I have any idea of your blessings or of your hopes—or of your regrets. You and I are being brought together by the dictates of a Universal Law, placed THERE long before us; to be There long after us...so much so that you can truly question to what extent do you and I even count, in the scheme of things?

I am moved to respond to the question. Yes, you matter; you are extremely important in the scheme of things. It is you who will set the reality for tomorrow. You will, by your actions—physical and mental, verbal and silent, hygienic and non-hygienic...you will make the right decisions. You will be the author of the future. From this day forward 'time' is placed in your hands. Use it as you think wise; share it as you are so moved; value it for every second it is worth, because God has given this to you—and to only you.

I am honored to have had this chance to speak with you, to communicate with you; to be the ears and eyes of the Agent who was told to interface with you. Now it is clear; you are a person of God.

23: IN SUMMARY

Stop, reduce, and minimize the poisoning of your body and mind. Do this by combining organic food choices [FVNS] with hygienic behaviors [Rules of Wellness]. This is a key part of your life-saving and life-preserving campaign.

Reduce the level of retained toxins. Engage recommended and professionally supervised 'detoxification procedures.' The primary, Natural Hygiene healing modality is therapeutic fasting (consuming pure water only for a minimum of three days) under professional guidance and/or instruction. Where fasting is not an option, then consume fresh squeezed juices, fruits-vegetables smoothies, and mono meals.

Flood' your body and mind with the best, most nurturing food and food-for-thought as might be available to you. Organically grown, raw fruits, vegetables, nuts, and seeds [FVNS™] are the most recommended foods on planet earth, from the perspective of the science of healthful living, Natural Hygiene.

Embrace and commit to implementing the 'rules of wellness' behaviors espoused by Natural Hygiene. These include positive mental activities, a variety of physical exercises, exposure to sunshine, fresh air, safe environments, calm and stress-free living atmosphere, much laughter and the fellowship of kindred spirits. Forgive yourself and forgive others, no matter what.

Remember the value of chewing—even your drinking water. Maintain your willingness to share with others the insights and inspiration you receive from the *www.OrganicWellnessCrusade.com* website. You are committing to a radical change in your lifestyle (assuming, of course, you are not now a Natural Hygienist)! The act of chewing can extend, even save your life. Chewing is, perhaps, the smartest way to enhance your health, now and in the future.

24: AFTER THOUGHT

The simple, yet profound strategy of the Science of Healthful Living has been articulated. I have given it to you in different ways, primarily in the same order: stop or reduce behaviors that pollute your body and mind; decrease the level of toxemia in your body and in your mind; feed your mind and body the healthiest 'foods' on planet earth; exercise and engage a positive lifestyle; re-learn how to chew your food until it liquefies; and forgive yourself and any others, for whatever.

The Common Cold: The 'common cold' is common (communal, universal, typical in many humans) because—by and large—they abuse their bodies in 'common' or similar ways.

When the body abuse ceases, the common cold ceases to be a factor of concern. Symptoms disappear. There is a 100% correlation between mind/body abuse and symptoms of the common cold. That is so because 'cold symptoms' are warnings, notifications that your body's 'pollution level' is near critical.

Suppose you ignored the 'cold symptoms.' What do you think would happen? For sure, your body/mind would become even more polluted, right? Now consider a long period during which even greater amounts of 'poisons' accumulate among and within your organs, tissues, and bodily functions—mental and physical.

Fast-forward 10, 20, 30, 40 years of accumulated toxic stuff housed and stored within your system. The evidence of this long-time storage—the 'cold' or 'disease' symptoms—are now given names and are treated as 'entities,' as something that has 'mysteriously' taken possession of or occupied your body or mind. The names given to 'these presumed invaders' describe both the location and the intensity of the dis-ease. If the irritation is in the guts, it is classified as stomach disease and is given a variety of names, depending upon intensity. This same pattern applies whether the distress is heart, lung, liver, kidney, brain, bladder, womb, prostate, head or feet.

The major point is that if allowed to continue to build up, one day the accumulated poisons would have become so critical an amount that Natural Hygienists would describe it as 'a crisis of toxemia,' while the medical establishment would call it a 'terminal cancer.'

So, now you know. Now you can see the picture: All the small amounts of toxic content your organism retains, down through the years, will dictate what 'illnesses' or 'disease' conditions you will deal with in your life. Nor does it change anything if you thought you were eating healthy and taking care of yourself. Poison in equals poison out.

Because there is no 'magic pill' that will cause you or me to change our unhealthy consumptive behaviors, nothing can protect us better than prevention. The degree to which the build-up of dis-ease is either prevented or significantly reduced will determine what illnesses, acute and chronic and degenerative 'dis-eases' you will experience during your lifetime.

Knowing what is stated above is good news! It is empowering; it confirms that it is possible to live life sickness-free, even in the industrialized multiplexes we call Chicago, New York, Philadelphia, Los Angeles, Boston, New Orleans, Houston, and Atlanta, etc. For sure, escaping industrial poisoning, you can better manage to control lethal amounts of dietary toxins. Natural Hygiene teaches such control.

Harvey and Marilyn Diamond's *Fit for Life,* a national Best Seller in the 1980's lays out the bigger hygienic story; my book, *Helping Hand:* 8-Day Diet Programs for People Who Care about Wellness, [Publius Publishing and Productions, Pacific Palisades, CA, 1986; *Helping Hand: A Guide to Healthy Living,* Beverly Publishers, Ltd., Oregun, Ikeja, Nigeria, 1990; Ihre Gesundheit liegt in Ihrer Hand, Waldthausen, Germany, 1992; *Helping Hand: Amerikan Daietto,* Tokai University Press, Tokyo, Japan, 1994] is a helpful guide for anyone wanting to transition from an animal-based to a plant-based dietary lifestyle. So, the story has been well told; it just has to be better implemented, to save more lives.

Actively practicing a hygienic lifestyle can prevent terminal disease from occurring. Or, it can offer realistic chances of slowing, if not reversing a set of circumstances which has been determined to be either 'a crisis of toxemia' or 'terminal cancer.' Whether the condition has already passed, or is approaching the point of no return, cannot be predicted; that can only be determined after the implementation of the hygienic lifestyle, doing so with a sense of urgency.

25: CONCLUDING STATEMENT

My prayer is that these words have not confused you, or wasted your time. Hopefully my words and thoughts have helped you sort through the many thoughts and questions and emotions you are dealing with. What has been written and shared has come from inspiration and personal belief. I would stake my own life on the counsel implied in all that is written herein.

If your level of internal pollution (toxemia) is and has been at the 'critical' level, for too long and has done too much internal damage, natural hygiene cannot promise remission. On the other hand, if your condition or the condition of someone you care about is still south of 'no return,' hygienic behaviors do offer realistic promise; and I urge you to consider making the commitment.

Finally, if you had pursued a natural hygienic lifestyle 10, 20, 30 years ago, you probably would not now be reading this small book. If you wish you had, not all is lost; you can share the book and its insight with someone you know who, if a change does not occur now, 10, 20, 30 years from today, that person could face a devastating pronouncement: 'Your condition is terminal.'

I am thankful to Almighty God for the revelation and insight I received back in 1986. I was 52, overweight and alcoholic, with various physical complaints and was beginning to notice my memory slipping away. A stranger I met on a plane to Carnival in Rio de Janeiro, Brazil later became a friend and introduced me to the science of Natural Hygiene. Now, at 82 years old, with not a single physical or mental complaint, I thank Ken and my God for the blessings! To show my appreciation, I do three things. I work out regularly and follow the Rules of Wellness; I pursue a raw, vegetarian lifestyle; and I will go any distance, at any hour to share my knowledge and commitment to the science of healthful living with anyone who asks me. I am also the creator, facilitator, writer, and website originator of *www.OrganicWellnessCrusade.com*.

Your donations may not be tax deductible, thank you.

Henry L. N. Anderson, Author
March 29, 2017

SUMMARY NOTATIONS

First, "cancer" is our code word. It stands for the 'cost' of industrialization. In other words, we all have "cancer cells" in us because that is 'the price' we pay for our modern society: the mass growth and marketing of food; the supplies of water, electricity, food and drink, clothing, housing, transportation, and all other amenities of modern living, including polluted air, the 'side effects' of all drugs-chemicals-medications-enrichment articles-adjustment articles, devices, and belief structures. These all extract a price, and that price is a reduction in a more pristine evolvement of our physical bodies, and of our mental actualities. So, visible cancer is our life-exchange price. The extent to which we actually pay depends upon many factors. For most of us, these are controllable factors. When we understand and manage the reality of 'mass production and distribution,' and undermine the negatives by our 'positive lifestyle,' we can and do escape the Reaper. And, we will never be diagnosed a cancer patient or victim. Cancer happens to many for one or two reasons—maybe three…or so. One, it is the 'cost of modern civilized co-existence.' Two, it results from an 'abusive' lifestyle. Three, cancer results from over (or intensive) exposure to industrialized components, like electrical radiation, vehicular exhaust/polluted air, personal habits of indulgence, and of course, a combination of these added to our individual 'belief structures.' What we believe is as important as what we physically consume.

Cancer is not 'the enemy;' it is the corresponding price generated by our other demands for a civilized, modern, industrialized existence in a developed society. Cancer, then, is 'our bodies' intake and management of internal pollution, with a wide-spread range of individual capacities to manage the poisons.

Stuff stored is toxic…no matter how 'little,' which by definition gets 'bigger' the older and more consuming is the individual. Each body reacts 'as it must' to the poisons it has been storing. And, by the way, 'cancer' is reversible (may be reduced, not eliminated) depending on how well one manages internal content—stored poisons (concentrated in the blood supply, but will 'next' where 'invited' by internal body flora or other conditions peculiar to one body as opposed to another.

A kind of 'cancer-like' abuse occurs in men, such that they birth children we label *autistic*. Why it is men who spawn the condition are men produce the chromosomes, which earlier, abusive lifestyles 'attacked,' killing off or weakening so many as to reduce 'normal' development (even though, in reality, there is no 'normal development' in industrialized societies). Of course, what is called 'normal' is a re-definition (which is what all diseases are). When a 'disease' is 'eliminated,' it is simply redefined (out of existence).

So, the question is: Will we ever be cancer-free (or find 'a cure for cancer')? You can answer that. And, the answer is: 'Of course not!' Nor will the 'research fund raising' ever stop either! Don't you get it?

ABOUT THE AUTHOR

Henry Lee Norman Brown Anderson was the fourth child born to Louise and Eggister Anderson, Washitaw descendants, in Ogeechee, Screven County, Georgia. He grew up in Savannah but left GA at the age of 16, headed for a new life in Philadelphia, Pennsylvania where he graduated from Benjamin Franklin High School for Boys, winning a Board of Education four-year scholarship to college.

He entered Earlham College in Richmond, Indiana as a pre-medical student, transferred and graduated from Cheyney University of Pennsylvania as a teacher. He was accepted as a candidate for the Episcopal priesthood by the Divinity School at Yale University, New Haven, CT., where in 1958, he met and became life-long friends with Rev. Dr. Martin Luther King, Jr., to whom 'a revelation' had him present a handwritten, 'John-the-Baptist' letter, advising Dr. King of his '…special reason for being on earth, and not to be distracted.…' Ten years from that meeting, Dr. King was assassinated in Memphis, Tennessee.

Arriving in Los Angeles on September 7, 1959 he later formed Western Publishers, Ltd., and was the first publisher ever to accept, finance, and publish a book (*She Walks in Beauty*, a novel) written by the famous 'Negro Historian,' J. A. Rogers. In 1960, he self-published his own first Small Book™, *You and Race: A Christian Reflects*. Years later he had a private audience with Mother Teresa *in* Calcutta, India, when she described Jesus' life mission in five words: 'Jesus did it unto them.'

In 1974, with some twenty family, friends, and students he co-founded City University Los Angeles, in response to the Carnegie Commission's Report that American higher education needed a system that would afford mature adults the opportunity to spend 'less time and more options' for completing a college degree. **CULA®** was accredited by the Empire Washitaw De Dugdahmoundyah and Empress Verdicee Turner-Goston. Later, Dr. Anderson was named Minister of Education by the Empress; and he and Dr. Margie N. Johnson, his wife represented the Empire Washitaw at the Indigenous Peoples Conference at the United Nations in Geneva, Switzerland in 2001. In the years immediately following, Dr. Anderson was appointed Chief Administrative Officer of Uaxashaktun (Empire Washitaw) De Dugdahmoundyah; and simultaneously, he was installed as a Judge for the Pembina Nation-- Little Shell Band of North America's Federal Tribal Circuit Court by Albert L. LaFontaine, Senior Judge for The Grand National Council of Confederated Nations, a Confederation of the United States Federal Government pursuant to the Treaty of 1778. Dr. Anderson was also appointed and served as Attorney General for the Pembina Nation – Little Shell Band of North Dakota.

In 1986, he was introduced to Natural Hygiene and became a vegetarian, later elevating to a fruitarian, and published his first book on 'the science of healthful living' in the same year. Now, some fourteen published books later, he gives us the present Small Book™, *HIDDEN HAND*, as a guide to coping with the mental terror and devastation of a medical doctor's pronouncement that 'you have cancer.' His hope, however, is that years before any such event, the public will have learned the content of this book, and all that is implied.

Dr. Anderson still works out regularly and follows the "Rules of Wellness." He is convinced that Natural Hygiene offers real hope and can be relied upon. He celebrates his "29th Birthday (for the 54th time!)" on May 23, 2017, with no medical complaints. When asked about his personal physician and medical treatments, he jokingly quips, "All my doctors are dead!"

And now, may *Love, Truth, Peace, Freedom, and Justice* guide your life.

Thank you for supporting:

www.OrganicWellnessCrusade.com. It helps save lives and assists in managing pain, confusion, frustration, and uncertainty, while providing a sound 'preventive' program as a proven and effective personal alternative for competing with terror at a personal level.

OTHER PUBLICATIONS BY THIS AUTHOR:

– *No Use Cryin'* (a novel about interracial love in Georgia in the 1950's), Western Publishers, LA, 1961

– *You and Race—A Christian Reflects*, 1960

– a.k.a.,Lee, Norhm, Ph.D., *Relationships, Truth, and Now,* American University Publishers, 2008

– *Revolutionary Urban Teaching,* 1972 UCLA doctoral dissertation by-product, 1973

– *African, Born in America,* Foreword by Dick Gregory, BLI Publishing, Beverly Hills, 1993

-"Foreword" in *The Diamond Sutra* by Wayne H. Huang, Translator, 1993

-"Publisher's Note" in *She Walks in Beauty*, first and only novel written by J. A. Rogers, 1963

-*Ihre Gesundheit liegt in Ihrer Hand,* Waldthausen, (Published in Germany),1992

-*A Guide to Healthy Living,* Beverly Publishers, Ikeja, Nigeria, West Africa, 1990

-*Helping Hand*, Japan Uni Agency, Inc., Noboru Miyaya, President,Tokyo, 1994

-*Organic Wellness Fasting Technique*, BLI Publishing, Beverly Hills, 1992

-*Mood Poetry for Everyone (In an Age of "Rap")*, Conquering Books, North Carolina, 2006

-*Helping Hand: 8-Day Diet Programs*, Publius Publishers, Pacific Palisades, CA, 1986

-*Nature and Purpose of Disease*, with T.C. Fry and Virginia Vetrano, Conquering Books, N.C., 2001

-*The N-WORD Revisited (Racism in 21st Century America),* Enigami & Rednow, N.Y.,1st Ed.,Jan 2017